# Longevity diet cook for seniors

*Make your choice to live and live up to 100 with 100 tasteful recipes just for you. Eat healthy to live healthy.*

Dr. Raymond Harris

# Table of content

# Introduction to Longevity Diets

In this section, we delve into the foundations of longevity diets, unraveling the principles that contribute to healthy aging. Recognizing the vital role nutrition plays in the lives of seniors, we explore how adopting a longevity-focused approach can enhance well-being and promote a fulfilling, active lifestyle. Join us on a journey to understand the symbiotic relationship between thoughtful dietary choices and the pursuit of a long, vibrant life for older individuals.

We'll unravel the science behind longevity diets, exploring the impact of nutrient-rich foods and their potential to support key aspects of senior health. Delving into the intricacies of aging, we'll shed light on how proper nutrition can influence longevity, energy levels, and resilience against age-related challenges. Let's embark on this exploration, discovering the significance of adopting a mindful and well-balanced approach to nutrition for seniors, ultimately paving the way for a healthier and more fulfilling aging journey.

## Understanding the principles of longevity diets

Longevity diets are rooted in the principles of promoting health, vitality,  and resilience as individuals age.  By understanding these principles, seniors can make informed dietary choices that contribute to overall well-being.  Nutrition plays a pivotal role in supporting physical functions, cognitive health,  and immune strength,  offering a powerful tool for maintaining quality of life in later years.  In this context, we'll explore how embracing the core tenets of longevity diets can empower seniors to lead healthier, more active lives, emphasizing the profound impact of nutrition on the aging process.

## Nutritional guideline for seniors

Seniors should focus on a well-balanced diet rich in nutrients. Emphasize:

1. Protein: Supports muscle health. Include lean meats,  poultry,  fish, eggs,  beans,  and dairy.

2.  Calcium and Vitamin D:Essential for bone health.  Dairy products,  leafy greens,  and fortified foods help.

3.  Fiber: Promotes digestive health. Whole grains,  fruits,  vegetables,  and legumes are good sources.

4.  Healthy Fats: Opt for sources like avocados,  nuts,  seeds,  and olive oil for heart health.

5. Hydration:Maintain adequate fluid intake, as dehydration risks increase with age.

6. Vitamins and Minerals:Ensure a variety of colorful fruits and vegetables for a spectrum of nutrients.

7. Limit Sodium and Sugar:Control salt intake to manage blood pressure, and minimize added sugars for overall health.

Always consult with a healthcare professional or nutritionist for personalized advice based on individual health needs.

# Benefit of nutritional food in terms of longevity in senior

Nutrient-rich foods play a crucial role in promoting longevity for seniors by offering several benefits:

1. Disease Prevention:A well-balanced diet can help prevent chronic diseases, such as heart disease, diabetes, and certain cancers, contributing to a longer, healthier life.

2. Immune Support:Proper nutrition supports a robust immune system, helping seniors fight off infections and illnesses more effectively.

3. Maintaining Healthy Weight:A balanced diet helps control weight, reducing the risk of obesity-related health issues and enhancing overall well-being.

4. Bone Health: Adequate calcium and vitamin D intake contribute to strong bones, reducing the risk of fractures and osteoporosis in later years.

5. Cognitive Function: Nutrient-rich foods, especially those high in antioxidants, may support brain health and reduce the risk of cognitive decline associated with aging.

6.  Muscle Maintenance: Adequate protein intake is vital for maintaining muscle mass,  strength,  and function, promoting mobility and independence.

7.  Heart Health: A diet low in saturated fats and rich in fruits,  vegetables,  and whole grains helps maintain cardiovascular health,  reducing the risk of heart-related issues.

8.  Digestive Health:A fiber-rich diet supports digestive health,  preventing constipation and other gastrointestinal issues common in aging.

9. Reduced Inflammation:Certain nutrients possess anti-inflammatory properties, helping to reduce inflammation linked to various age-related diseases.

Remember, individual nutritional needs can vary, and it's essential to tailor dietary choices to specific health conditions and preferences. Regular check-ups with healthcare professionals can guide seniors toward a diet that supports longevity and overall well-being.

# Things to do to aid their lives

Seniors can enhance their lives by incorporating various activities:

1. Stay Active:Engage in regular physical activity like walking, swimming,  or gentle exercises to maintain mobility and overall health.

2.  Socialize: Foster social connections through clubs,  community groups,  or spending time with family and friends, which can positively impact mental and emotional well-being.

3. Hobbies:Pursue hobbies or learn new ones to stay mentally stimulated and enjoy fulfilling activities.

4. Mindfulness Practices: Practice mindfulness, meditation, or yoga to promote relaxation and reduce stress.

5. Volunteer:Contribute to the community by volunteering, offering skills and experience, which can provide a sense of purpose.

6. Regular Health Check-ups:Schedule routine health check-ups to monitor and address any health concerns promptly.

7. Stay Mentally Active:Engage in activities that challenge the mind, such as puzzles, games, or reading, to support cognitive function.

8. Healthy Eating:Adopt a balanced and nutritious diet to support overall health and well-being.

9. Adaptive Technologies:Embrace technology and gadgets that can simplify daily tasks, making life more comfortable.

10. Safety Measures: Implement safety measures at home,

such as removing tripping hazards and ensuring proper lighting,  to prevent accidents.

11.  Stay Informed: Stay informed about community resources,  support services,  and programs available for seniors.

Remember,  individual preferences and health conditions vary,  so tailor activities to personal interests and needs.  Regular communication with healthcare professionals can provide guidance on maintaining a healthy and fulfilling lifestyle in the senior years.

# Chapter two

## Exercise role in life longevity for seniors

Regular exercise plays a crucial role in promoting longevity for seniors by offering various benefits:

1. Maintains Mobility: Regular physical activity helps preserve joint flexibility and muscle strength,  contributing to overall mobility and independence.

2.  Heart Health: Exercise improves cardiovascular health,

reducing the risk of heart disease and related issues, which can impact longevity.

3. Bone Health: Weight-bearing exercises, such as walking or resistance training, support bone density, reducing the risk of fractures and osteoporosis.

4. Cognitive Function:Physical activity is linked to better cognitive function, potentially reducing the risk of cognitive decline and dementia in later years.

5. Balances Weight: Regular exercise helps manage weight,

reducing the risk of obesity-related conditions that can affect overall health and lifespan.

6.  Improves  Mood:Physical activity stimulates the release of endorphins, promoting a positive mood and reducing the risk of depression and anxiety.

7.  Enhances Sleep:Regular exercise can contribute to better sleep quality, which is vital for overall health and well-being.

8.  Manages Chronic Conditions: Exercise can help manage chronic

conditions such as diabetes, arthritis, and hypertension, contributing to a longer, healthier life.

9. Boosts Immunity:Physical activity supports a robust immune system, helping seniors fend off illnesses and infections.

10. Social Engagement:Participating in group exercises or activities promotes social connections, which can positively impact mental and emotional well-being.

It's crucial to tailor exercise routines to individual capabilities and health conditions.

Consulting with healthcare professionals or fitness experts can help seniors design a safe and effective exercise plan that aligns with their specific needs and goals.

# Chapter three

## breakfast recipes

1. Classic Oatmeal:
   Ingredients:
     1 cup rolled oats
     2 cups milk (or water)
     Toppings: berries, nuts, honey
   Instructions:
     1. Boil oats in milk or water.
     2. Simmer until desired consistency.
     3. Top with berries, nuts, and a
drizzle of honey.

2.  Avocado Toast:
    Ingredients:
      1 slice whole-grain bread
      1 ripe avocado
      Salt, pepper, red pepper flakes
    Instructions:
      1.  Toast the bread.
      2.  Mash avocado and spread on toast.
      3.  Sprinkle with salt, pepper, and
red pepper flakes.

 3.  Greek Yogurt Parfait:
    Ingredients:
      1 cup Greek yogurt
      Granola
      Mixed berries
      Honey
    Instructions:

1. Layer yogurt, granola, and berries.
2. Repeat layers.
3. Drizzle with honey.

4. Spinach and Feta Omelette:
Ingredients:
  2 eggs
  Handful of spinach
  Feta cheese
  Salt, pepper
Instructions:
  1. Whisk eggs and pour into a hot pan.
  2. Add spinach and feta.
  3. Fold into an omelette; season with salt and pepper.

5.  Smoothie Bowl:
   Ingredients:
    1 frozen banana
    1/2 cup berries
    1/2 cup almond milk
    Toppings: granola,  chia seeds
   Instructions:
    1.  Blend banana,  berries,  and
almond milk.
    2.  Pour into a bowl; top with granola
and chia seeds.

6.  Pancakes:
Ingredients:
    1 cup flour
   1 tbsp sugar
   1 tsp baking powder
    1 egg

3/4 cup milk
Instructio&hnsn:
1. Mix dry ingredients; add egg and milk.
2. Cook spoonfuls of batter on a griddle.

7. Chia Seed Pudding:
Ingredients:
2 tbsp chia seeds
1 cup milk (any type)
1 tsp vanilla extract
Fresh fruit
Instructions:
1. Mix chia seeds, milk, and vanilla.
2. Refrigerate overnight; top with fruit.

8.  Vegetable Breakfast Burrito:
    Ingredients:
      1 whole-grain tortilla
      Scrambled eggs
      Black beans, salsa, avocado
    Instructions:
      1. Fill tortilla with scrambled eggs,
beans, salsa, and avocado.
      2. Roll into a burrito.

  9.  Peanut Butter Banana Toast:
    Ingredients:
      1 slice whole-grain bread
      Peanut butter
      Sliced banana
    Instructions:
      1. Toast the bread.

2.  Spread peanut butter and top with banana slices.

10.  Egg and Veggie Muffins:
   Ingredients:
   Eggs
   Chopped vegetables (bell peppers, spinach)
   Salt, pepper, cheese
   Instructions:
   1.  Whisk eggs; mix with veggies, salt, pepper.
   2.  Pour into muffin tin; bake until set.

Adjust quantities based on personal preferences,  and enjoy your nutritious breakfast!

## lunch

1.  Grilled Chicken Salad:
   Ingredients:
      Grilled chicken breast
      Mixed greens
      Cherry tomatoes
      Cucumber
      Balsamic vinaigrette
    Instructions:
    1.  Slice grilled chicken and arrange on a bed of mixed greens.

2. Add cherry tomatoes and
cucumber.
3. Drizzle with balsamic vinaigrette.

2. Quinoa Bowl with Roasted
Vegetables:
Ingredients:
Cooked quinoa
Roasted vegetables (e. g. , bell
peppers, zucchini)
Chickpeas
Feta cheese
Instructions:
1. Combine quinoa, roasted
vegetables, and chickpeas in a bowl.
2. Top with crumbled feta.

3.  Vegetarian Wrap:
   Ingredients:
     Whole-grain wrap
     Hummus
     Avocado slices
     Shredded lettuce
     Sliced bell peppers
   Instructions:
     1.  Spread hummus on the wrap.
     2.  Layer with avocado, lettuce, and
bell peppers.
     3.  Roll it up and slice.

4.  Salmon and Quinoa Salad:
   Ingredients:
     Grilled salmon fillet
     Quinoa
     Spinach

Mango chunks
Lemon-tahini dressing
Instructions:
1.  Flake salmon over a bed of quinoa and spinach.
2.  Add mango chunks.
3.  Drizzle with lemon-tahini dressing.

5.  Mushroom and Spinach Omelette:
Ingredients:
Eggs
Sliced mushrooms
Spinach
Feta cheese
Instructions:
1.  Whisk eggs and pour into a hot pan.

2.  Add mushrooms, spinach, and feta.

3.  Fold into an omelette.


6.  Chickpea and Vegetable Stir-Fry:
Ingredients:
Chickpeas
Broccoli florets
Bell peppers
Soy sauce
Brown rice
Instructions:
1.  Stir-fry chickpeas and vegetables in soy sauce.

2.  Serve over cooked brown rice.


7.  Caprese Sandwich:
Ingredients:

Whole-grain bread
Mozzarella cheese
Tomato slices
Fresh basil leaves
Balsamic glaze
Instructions:
1. Layer mozzarella, tomato, and basil on bread.
2. Drizzle with balsamic glaze.

8. Lentil Soup:
Ingredients:
Lentils
Carrots
Celery
Vegetable broth
Spinach
Instructions:

1. Cook lentils, carrots, and celery in vegetable broth.

2. Add spinach before serving.

9. Turkey and Avocado Wrap:
Ingredients:
   Turkey slices
   Whole-grain wrap
   Avocado
   Lettuce
   Greek yogurt dressing

Instructions:
   1. Layer turkey, avocado, and lettuce on the wrap.

   2. Drizzle with Greek yogurt dressing.

10.  Vegetable and Chickpea Curry:
   Ingredients:
   Chickpeas
   Mixed vegetables (e. g. ,  cauliflower, peas)
   Curry sauce
   Brown rice
   Instructions:
   1.  Simmer chickpeas and vegetables in curry sauce.
   2.  Serve over cooked brown rice.

Feel free to customize these recipes based on your preferences and dietary needs.  Enjoy your nutritious lunches!

# Dinner

1. Baked Lemon Garlic Chicken:
Ingredients:
    Chicken breasts
    Lemon
     Garlic cloves
    Olive oil
     Rosemary

Instructions:
    1.  Marinate chicken in a mixture of lemon juice,  minced garlic,  olive oil, and rosemary.
    2.  Bake until fully cooked.

2.  Vegetarian Stir-Fried Noodles:
   Ingredients:
     Egg noodles
     Tofu or tempeh
     Mixed vegetables (bell peppers,
broccoli)
     Soy sauce
   Instructions:
     1.  Stir-fry tofu/tempeh and
vegetables.
     2.  Toss with cooked egg noodles and
soy sauce.

3. Salmon with Roasted Vegetables:
   Ingredients:
     Salmon fillets
     Sweet potatoes

Brussels sprouts
Olive oil
Dill
Instructions:
1. Roast salmon and vegetables with olive oil and dill until cooked.

4. Quinoa and Black Bean Stuffed Peppers:
Ingredients:
Bell peppers
Quinoa
Black beans
Corn
Salsa
Instructions:

1.  Mix cooked quinoa,  black beans, corn,  and salsa.
2.  Stuff the mixture into halved bell peppers; bake.

5.  Shrimp and Broccoli Stir-Fry:
    Ingredients:
      Shrimp
      Broccoli florets
      Soy sauce
      Ginger
      Garlic
    Instructions:
    1.  Stir-fry shrimp and broccoli with soy sauce,  ginger,  and garlic.

6. Mushroom Risotto:
    Ingredients:

Arborio rice
Mushrooms
Onion
Vegetable broth
Parmesan cheese
Instructions:
1. Sauté  mushrooms and onions; add rice.
2. Gradually add vegetable broth; stir until creamy.
3. Top with Parmesan cheese.

7. Grilled Veggie and Chicken Skewers:
Ingredients:
Chicken chunks
Cherry tomatoes
Zucchini

Red onion
Olive oil,  herbs
Instructions:
1. Thread chicken and vegetables onto skewers.
2. Grill until chicken is cooked.

8. Eggplant Parmesan:
Ingredients:
Eggplant slices
Marinara sauce
Mozzarella cheese
Parmesan cheese
Basil
Instructions:
1. Layer eggplant with marinara, mozzarella,  and Parmesan; bake.

2.  Garnish with fresh basil.

 9.  Teriyaki Tofu and Vegetable
Stir-Fry:
   Ingredients:
     Tofu
     Mixed vegetables (bell peppers,
snow peas)
     Teriyaki sauce
     Brown rice
   Instructions:
     1.  Stir-fry tofu and vegetables with
teriyaki sauce.
     2.  Serve over cooked brown rice.

10.  Chickpea and Spinach Curry:
   Ingredients:
    Chickpeas

Spinach

Coconut milk

Curry spices

Basmati rice

Instructions:

1. Simmer chickpeas and spinach in coconut milk with curry spices.

2. Serve over cooked basmati rice.

Adjust these recipes based on your preferences and dietary needs. Enjoy your delicious dinners!

healthy snack ideas along with their ingredients and instructions:

1. Greek Yogurt with Berries:
   Ingredients:
     Greek yogurt
     Mixed berries (blueberries, strawberries)
     Honey
   Instructions:
     1.  Spoon Greek yogurt into a bowl.
     2.  Top with fresh berries and drizzle with honey.

2.  Apple Slices with Almond Butter:
   Ingredients:
    Apple slices
    Almond butter
   Instructions:
    1.  Spread almond butter on apple slices.

3.  Vegetable Sticks with Hummus:
   Ingredients:
    Carrot, cucumber, and bell pepper sticks
    Hummus
   Instructions:
    1.  Dip vegetable sticks into hummus.

4. Trail Mix:
  Ingredients:
    Mixed nuts (almonds, walnuts)
    Dried fruits (raisins, apricots)
    Dark chocolate chips
  Instructions:
    1. Mix nuts, dried fruits, and dark chocolate.

5. Hard-Boiled Eggs:
  Ingredients:
    Hard-boiled eggs
    Salt, pepper
  Instructions:
    1. Sprinkle eggs with salt and pepper.

6. Cottage Cheese with Pineapple:
  Ingredients:

Cottage cheese
Fresh pineapple chunks
Instructions:
1. Combine cottage cheese and pineapple.

7. Whole Grain Crackers with Cheese:
Ingredients:
Whole grain crackers
Cheese slices
Instructions:
1. Pair crackers with cheese slices.

8. Smoothie:
Ingredients:
Banana
Spinach
Greek yogurt

Almond milk
Instructions:
1. Blend banana, spinach, Greek yogurt, and almond milk.

9. Popcorn with Nutritional Yeast:
Ingredients:
Air-popped popcorn
Nutritional yeast
Olive oil
Instructions:
1. Drizzle popcorn with olive oil and sprinkle with nutritional yeast.

10. Avocado Toast with Cherry Tomatoes:
Ingredients:
Whole-grain toast

Avocado
Cherry tomatoes
Salt,  pepper
Instructions:
1.  Spread mashed avocado on toast.
2.  Top with halved cherry tomatoes; season with salt and pepper.

These snacks are not only tasty but also provide a mix of nutrients to keep you energized throughout the day.  Adjust portion sizes to fit your dietary preferences and needs.  Enjoy your healthy snacks!

soup and stew recipes with their ingredients and instructions:

1. Chicken Noodle Soup:
   Ingredients:
     Chicken broth
     Cooked chicken
     Carrots, celery, and onion
     Egg noodles
   Instructions:
     1. Simmer vegetables and chicken in broth.
     2. Add cooked noodles before serving.

2. Vegetarian Lentil Soup:
   Ingredients:

Green lentils

Carrots, celery, and onion

Vegetable broth

Cumin, coriander, and thyme

Instructions:

1. Cook lentils and vegetables in broth.

2. Season with cumin, coriander, and thyme.

3. Beef and Vegetable Stew:

Ingredients:

Beef stew meat

Potatoes, carrots, and peas

Beef broth

Tomato paste

Instructions:

1.  Brown beef; add vegetables,  broth, and tomato paste.

2.  Simmer until meat is tender.

4.  Butternut Squash Soup:
   Ingredients:
     Butternut squash
     Onion and garlic
     Vegetable broth
     Nutmeg and cinnamon
   Instructions:
     1.  Roast squash,  onion,  and garlic.
     2.  Blend with broth; season with nutmeg and cinnamon.

5.  Minestrone Soup:
   Ingredients:
     Cannellini beans

Pasta

Tomatoes, carrots, and spinach

Vegetable broth

Instructions:

1. Simmer beans, pasta, vegetables, and broth.

2. Add spinach before serving.

6. Tomato Basil Soup:

Ingredients:

Tomatoes

Onion and garlic

Vegetable broth

Fresh basil

Instructions:

1. Sauté onion and garlic; add tomatoes and broth.

2. Blend; stir in fresh basil.

7. Chickpea and Spinach Stew:
   Ingredients:
     Chickpeas
     Spinach
     Tomatoes and carrots
     Vegetable broth
   Instructions:
   1. Simmer chickpeas, spinach, vegetables, and broth.
   2. Season to taste.

8. Potato Leek Soup:
   Ingredients:
     Potatoes and leeks
     Chicken or vegetable broth
     Butter and cream

Instructions:
1.  Sauté leeks and potatoes in butter.
2.  Add broth; blend until smooth. Stir in cream.

9.  Chicken and Wild Rice Soup:
    Ingredients:
     Cooked chicken
     Wild rice
     Carrots, celery, and onion
     Chicken broth
    Instructions:
    1.  Simmer vegetables, chicken, rice, and broth.

10.  Moroccan Lentil Stew:
    Ingredients:
     Red lentils

Sweet potatoes and carrots

Chickpeas

Moroccan spices (cumin, coriander, cinnamon)

Instructions:

1. Cook lentils, sweet potatoes, carrots, and chickpeas in broth.

2. Season with Moroccan spices.

These recipes offer a variety of flavors and ingredients, providing nutritious and comforting options for soups and stews. Adjust ingredients and seasoning based on personal preferences and dietary needs. Enjoy these hearty and flavorful dishes!

salad recipes with their components
and instructions:

1. Classic Caesar Salad: Ingredients:
   Romaine lettuce
   Caesar dressing
   Croutons Parmesan cheese
  Instructions:
   1.  Toss chopped lettuce with Caesar
dressing.
   2.  Add croutons and shaved
Parmesan.

 2.  Caprese Salad: Ingredients:
Tomatoes
   Fresh mozzarella

Fresh basil
Balsamic glaze
Instructions:
1.  Arrange tomato and mozzarella slices.
2.  Garnish with fresh basil; sprinkle with balsamic glaze.

3.  Greek Salad: Ingredients: Cucumber, tomatoes,  and red onion
Feta cheese
Kalamata olives
Olive oil with oregano
Instructions:
1.  Combine chopped veggies,  olives, and feta.

2.  Drizzle with olive oil; sprinkle with oregano.

4.  Quinoa and Avocado Salad:
Ingredients:
    Cooked quinoa
    Avocado
    Cherry tomatoes
    Cilantro
    Lime dressing
   Instructions:
   1.  Mix quinoa, avocado, tomatoes, and cilantro.
   2.  Toss with lime dressing.

5. Kale and Cranberry Salad:
Ingredients:
    Kale

Dried cranberries
 Pecans
 Feta cheese
 Balsamic vinaigrette
Instructions:
  1.  Massage kale with balsamic
vinaigrette.
  2.  Add cranberries, pecans, and
crumbled feta.

6.  Asian Sesame Chicken Salad:
Ingredients:
  Grilled chicken
 Mixed greens
  Mandarin oranges
  Sesame dressing
  Chow mein noodles
 Instructions:

1.  Toss greens, chicken, and mandarin oranges.

2.  Drizzle with sesame dressing; top with chow mein noodles.


7.  Spinach and Strawberry Salad:
Ingredients:
  Baby spinach
  Sliced strawberries
  Goat cheese
  Balsamic vinaigrette
Instructions:

1.  Combine spinach, strawberries, and goat cheese.

2.  Drizzle with balsamic vinaigrette.

8.  Mango and Black Bean Salad:
Ingredients:
    Black beans
    Mango
    Red onion
    Cilantro
    Lime dressing
  Instructions:
    1.  Mix black beans,  diced mango,
chopped onion,  and cilantro.
    2.  Toss with lime dressing.


 9.  Tuna Nicoise Salad: Ingredients:
    Tuna
    Mixed greens
    Cherry tomatoes
    Hard-boiled eggs

Kalamata olives

Instructions:

1. Arrange greens, tuna, tomatoes, eggs, and olives.

2. Drizzle with your choice of dressing.


10. Couscous and Vegetable Salad:

Ingredients:

Cooked couscous Bell peppers, cucumber, and cherry tomatoes

Feta cheese

Lemon vinaigrette

Instructions:

1. Combine couscous, chopped veggies, and feta.

2. Toss with lemon vinaigrette.

These salad dishes give a blend of tastes and textures, making them delightful and healthful. Adjust ingredients and dressings according on personal tastes. Enjoy these delicious salads!

## dessert recipes with their components and instructions:

1. Classic Chocolate Chip Cookies:
Ingredients:
    Butter, sugar, and brown sugar
    Eggs Vanilla extract

Flour, baking soda, salt
Chocolate chips
Instructions:
1. Cream butter and sugars. Add eggs and vanilla.
2. Mix in dry ingredients; mix in chocolate chips.
3. Drop spoonfuls onto a baking sheet; bake until brown.

2. Homemade Apple Crisp: Ingredients:
Apples
Brown sugar
Flour, oats, and butter
Cinnamon and nutmeg
Instructions:
1. Mix sliced apples with sugar and spices.

2.  Combine flour,  oats,  and butter for the topping.

3.  Bake till bubbling and golden.


3.  Strawberry Shortcake: Ingredients:
Fresh strawberries

Shortcakes or sponge cake

Whipped cream

Instructions:

1.  Slice strawberries and sweeten if required.

2.  Layer strawberries and whipped cream between shortcakes.


4.  Chocolate Avocado Mousse:
Ingredients:

Ripe avocados

Cocoa powder

Maple syrup
Vanilla extract
Instructions:
1. Blend avocados, cocoa powder, maple syrup, and vanilla until smooth.
2. Chill before serving.

5. Lemon Bars:
Ingredients:
Shortbread crust
Eggs, sugar, and flour
Lemon juice with zest
Instructions:
1. Mix ingredients; pour over cooked crust.
2. Bake until firm; cool before cutting into bars.

6.  Banana Bread: Ingredients:
    Ripe bananas
    Sugar,  eggs,  and butter
    Flour,  baking soda,  and salt
   Instructions:
    1.  Mash bananas; blend with sugar,
eggs,  and melted butter.
    2.  Stir in dry ingredients; bake until a
toothpick comes out clean.

 7.  Peach Cobbler: Ingredients: Fresh or
canned peaches
    Sugar Flour,  baking powder,  and
salt
    Milk
   Instructions:
    1.  Mix peaches and sugar; let settle.

2.  Combine flour, baking powder, salt, and milk for the batter.

3.  Pour batter over peaches; bake until golden.

8.  Raspberry Cheesecake Bars:
Ingredients:
  Graham cracker crust
  Cream cheese, sugar, and eggs
  Raspberry jam
Instructions:
1.  Beat cream cheese, sugar, and eggs.

2.  Pour over crust; swirl in raspberry jam.

3.  Bake until firm; cool before slicing.

9.  Coconut Rice Pudding: Ingredients:
    Cooked rice
    Coconut milk
    Sugar with vanilla extract
    Cinnamon
   Instructions:
   1.  Simmer rice, coconut milk, sugar, and vanilla until smooth.
   2.  Sprinkle with cinnamon before serving.

10.  Cherry Chocolate Tart: Ingredients:
    Chocolate cookie crust
    Dark chocolate ganache
    Fresh cherries
   Instructions:
   1.  Fill the crust with chocolate ganache.

2. Top with pitted cherries; cool before slicing.

These dessert dishes provide a range of tastes and textures. Adjust ingredients depending on tastes and dietary requirements. Enjoy these tasty goodies!

## veggie dishes with their components and instructions:

1. Roasted veggies: Ingredients:
Assorted veggies (carrots, bell peppers, zucchini)
    Olive oil

Garlic, minced
Herbs (rosemary, thyme)
Instructions:
1. Toss veggies with olive oil, garlic, and herbs.
2. Roast in the oven until tender.

2. Stir-Fried Broccoli and Tofu:
Ingredients:
Broccoli florets
Firm tofu, cubed
Soy sauce
Ginger with garlic, minced
Sesame oil
Instructions:

1. Stir-fry tofu and broccoli in sesame oil.

2. Add soy sauce, ginger, and garlic.

3. Zucchini Noodles with Pesto:
Ingredients: Zucchini, spiralized
Cherry tomatoes, halved Pesto sauce
Pine nuts
Instructions:

1. Sauté zucchini noodles; add tomatoes.

2. Toss with pesto; sprinkle pine nuts.

4. Mushroom Risotto: Ingredients:
Arborio rice
Mushrooms, sliced onion and garlic, minced Vegetable broth Parmesan cheese

Instructions:
   1.  Sauté mushrooms,  onion,  and garlic.
   2.  Add rice; gradually add broth.  Stir in Parmesan.

5.  Grilled Eggplant with Balsamic Glaze:
   Ingredients: Eggplant,  sliced Olive oil
   Balsamic glaze
   Fresh basil
  Instructions:
   1.  Brush eggplant with olive oil; grill.
   2.  Drizzle with balsamic glaze; garnish with basil.

6.  Cauliflower Buffalo Bites:
   Ingredients:

Cauliflower florets
 Buffalo sauce
 Greek yogurt or ranch dressing
Instructions:
 1. Coat cauliflower in buffalo sauce; bake.
 2. Serve with Greek yogurt or ranch.

7. Brussels Sprouts Salad:
 Ingredients:
  Shredded Brussels sprouts
  Dried cranberries
  Almonds
  Feta cheese
  Balsamic vinaigrette
 Instructions:

1. Combine shredded Brussels sprouts, cranberries, almonds, and feta.

2. Toss with balsamic vinaigrette.

8. Sweet Potato and Chickpea Curry:
    Ingredients:
      Sweet potatoes, diced Chickpeas
      Coconut milk
      Curry spices
      Spinach
    Instructions:
    1. Simmer sweet potatoes and chickpeas in coconut milk.

2. Add curry spices; toss in spinach.

9. Tomato and Cucumber Salad:
Ingredients: Tomatoes, diced
Cucumber, sliced Red onion, thinly
sliced Olive oil and red wine vinegar
   Fresh herbs (parsley, dill)
Instructions:
   1. Combine tomatoes, cucumber,
and red onion.
   2. Dress with olive oil, red wine
vinegar, and herbs.

10. Spaghetti Squash Primavera:
   Ingredients:
     Spaghetti squash, roasted
     Mixed veggies (bell peppers, cherry
tomatoes)

Olive oil

Garlic,  minced

Instructions:

1.  Sauté mixed veggies in olive oil and garlic.

2.  Toss with roasted spaghetti squash.

These vegetable dishes provide a range of tastes and techniques.  Adjust ingredients depending on tastes and dietary requirements.

www.ingramcontent.com/pod-product-compliance
Lightning Source LLC
Chambersburg PA
CBHW061005260726
48661CB00005B/2056